Pressure Co
Cookbook for Busy People

Tasty and Easy Recipes to Prepare in
your Electric Pressure Cooker

Maria Marshal

Table Of Contents

BREAKFAST RECIPES

Peach and Cottage Breakfast

(Ready in about 20 minutes | Servings 4)

Ingredients

1. 4 peaches, pitted and halved

1. 1/4 cup water

1. 1/4 cup apple juice

1. 1/4 teaspoon vanilla extract

1. 2 tablespoons brown sugar

1. 1/8 teaspoon grated nutmeg

1. 1/4 teaspoon ground cinnamon

1. 1 cup cottage cheese

1. 2 tablespoons maple syrup

Directions

1. Add all the above ingredients, except for cottage cheese, to your pressure cooker. Securely lock the lid and cook on LOW for 4 to 5 minutes.
2. Release pressure, and adjust the seasonings. Remove peaches from the cooker and reserve.

3. Combine cottage cheese with maple syrup.

4. To serve: place one peach on each serving plate. Serve topped with a dollop of cheese mixture. Enjoy!

Quick and Easy Aromatic Oatmeal

(Ready in about 10 minutes | Servings 4)

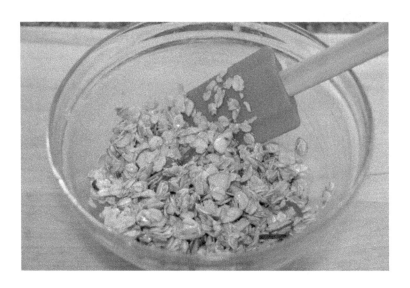

Ingredients

1. 3 tablespoons butter

1. 1 cup steel-cut oats

1. 3 ½ cups water

1. 1/4 teaspoon grated nutmeg

1. 1/2 teaspoon ground cinnamon

1. A pinch of salt

1. 1/4 cup low-fat milk

1. 1/4 cup light brown sugar

Directions

1. Warm butter on HIGH until melted.

2. Then, add the steel-cut oats, water, grated nutmeg, cinnamon, and salt. Seal the cooker's lid and cook under HIGH pressure for 5 minutes.

3. Next, release pressure and uncover. Add the milk and brown sugar; stir tocombine and serve right away.

Fruit Steel-Cut Oats

(Ready in about 25 minutes | Servings 6)

Ingredients

1. 1 ½ cups steel-cut oats

1. 1/2 cup dates, chopped

1. 1/2 cup dried currants

1. 3 apples, cored and diced

1. 1 teaspoon pumpkin pie spice

1. 6 cups water

1. 1 cup soy milk

Directions

1. Prepare the ingredients according to the manufacturer's directions. Then,transfer them to a pressure cooker.

2. Now set your cooker to HIGH and cook for 18 minutes.

3. Sweeten with some honey if desired. Enjoy!

14

FAST SNACKS RECIPES
Bacon and Bean Dip
(Ready in about 30 minutes | Servings 12)

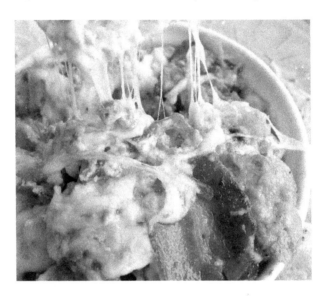

Ingredients

1. 2 cups water

1. 1 cup dried beans

1. 4 slices bacon, finely diced

1. 2 cloves garlic, peeled and minced

1. 1 onion, peeled and diced

1. 1 (14 ½-ounce) can tomatoes, diced
1. 2 teaspoons chili powder

1. 1/2 teaspoon dried basil

1. Sea salt and black pepper, to taste

1. 1/4 cup fresh parsley, finely chopped

1. 1 cup sharp cheese, grated

1. Avocado slices, for garnish

Directions

1. Add the water and beans to a container and let it soak overnight. Drain thebeans and set aside.

2. Throw the bacon, garlic, and onion into your cooker. Sauté for 3 to 4minutes or until the onions are translucent.

3. Then, stir the beans into the pressure cooker together with the tomatoes, chili powder, and basil. Lock the lid into place. Bring to HIGH pressure andmaintain pressure for 12 minutes.

4. Turn off the heat and allow pressure to release for 10 minutes. Uncover andtransfer the prepared bean mixture to your food processor.

Add the sea salt,black pepper, and parsley and blend until smooth.

5. Transfer the dip to a fondue pot and add cheese. Stir to combine andgarnish with avocado. Serve immediately with your favorite dippers.

Caribbean-Style Relish

(Ready in about 30 minutes | Servings 12)

Ingredients

1. 7 cups water

1. 1 ½ cups kidney beans

1. 2 teaspoons olive oil

1. Salt and ground black pepper, to taste

1. 2 tablespoons tahini paste

1. 1/4 cup pineapple, drained and crushed

1. 1/2 teaspoon dried cumin

1. 1 teaspoon garlic powder

1. 1/2 cup fresh cilantro, finely minced

Directions

1. Add 3 cups of water and kidney beans to your cooker; let it soak overnight. Drain and replace to the pressure cooker. Pour in the remaining 4 cups ofwater. Add the olive oil and lock the lid into place.

2. Bring to HIGH pressure and maintain this pressure for 10 to 15 minutes.Remove from the heat. Then, quick release any remaining pressure.

3. Add the cooked beans to the bowl of your blender or a food processor. Stirin the rest of the above ingredients and pulse until it is well combined but still a little chunky.

4. Place in a refrigerator to chill, and serve as a dip for chips if desired.

Glazed Carrots with Cranberries

(Ready in about 5 minutes | Servings 6)

Ingredients

1. 1 cup water

1. 2 pounds carrots, sliced diagonally

1. 1/4 cup dried cranberries

1. A pinch of kosher salt

1. 3/4 teaspoon black pepper

1. 2 tablespoons butter

1. 2 tablespoons maple syrup

Directions

1. Put the water, carrots, and cranberries into the pressure cooker. Close the lid of the cooker. Cook for 3 to 4 minutes at LOW pressure.

2. While the carrots are still warm, add the salt, black pepper, butter, and maple syrup. Gently stir to combine. Serve right now.

LUNCH RECIPES
Creamed Sausage and Spinach Soup
(Ready in about 20 minutes | Servings 6)

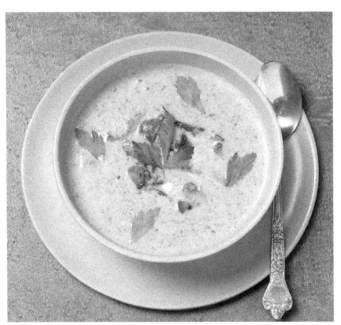

Ingredients

1. 2 tablespoons vegetable oil

1. 1 pound ground sausage

1. 3 cloves garlic, peeled and minced

1. 1 onion, peeled and diced

1. 6 cups chicken broth

1. 1 (10-ounce) bag spinach leaves

1. 4 carrots, thickly sliced

1. 1 teaspoon sugar

1. 1 teaspoon dried basil

1. 1 teaspoon dried oregano

1. 1/4 teaspoon red pepper flakes, crushed

1. Salt and ground black pepper, to taste

1. 1/2 cup heavy cream

Directions

1. First of all, heat vegetable oil until sizzling. Then, sauté the sausage, garlicand onion, until the sausage is browned, the onion is translucent, and thegarlic is fragrant.

2. Add the rest of the ingredients, except for heavy cream.

3. Securely lock the lid and set on HIGH for 3 minutes. Then, release thecooker's pressure.

4. Add heavy cream before serving and enjoy!

Satisfying Chicken and Rice Soup

(Ready in about 30 minutes | Servings 6)

Ingredients

1. 1 pound chicken thighs, boneless, skinless and cubed

1. 3 tablespoons flour

1. Salt and ground black pepper, to taste

1. 3 tablespoons butter

1. 1 tablespoon canola oil

1. 1 onion, diced

1. 2 large carrots, chopped

1. 2 large stalks celery, chopped

1. 2 tablespoons tomato paste

1. 1 rosemary sprig

1. 1 thyme spring

1. 1 ¼ cups wild rice

1. 6 cups chicken broth

1. 1 cup heavy cream

Directions

1. Coat the chicken thighs with sifted flour; season with salt and black pepper.

2. Now, heat butter and canola oil on HIGH until melted.

3. Lay the prepared chicken at the bottom of the pressure cooker; cook untilthey are lightly browned, about 5 minutes.

4. Add the rest of the ingredients, except for heavy cream; cook for 12 to 14minutes on HIGH.

5. Let the pressure release naturally and gradually. Add heavy cream, and stirto combine. Serve warm.

Cheese and Onion Soup

(Ready in about 20 minutes | Servings 6)

Ingredients

1. 3 tablespoons butter

1. 2 onions, peeled and thinly sliced

1. 2 teaspoons sugar

1. 5 cups beef broth

1. 2 tablespoons red wine

1. 1 bay leaf

1. 1 teaspoon dried thyme

1. Sea salt and freshly ground black pepper

1. 6 slices Provolone cheese

Directions

1. In your pressure cooker, warm butter on HIGH until sizzling.

2. Cook the onions and sugar in the cooker, until they are caramelized, forabout 10 minutes.

3. Add the beef broth, wine, bay leaf, dried thyme, salt, and ground black pepper; stir to combine. Now lock the pressure cooker's lid and cook for 8to 10 minutes on HIGH.

4. Ladle into soup bowls and top with Provolone cheese. Serve and enjoy!

Rich Garbanzo Bean Soup

(Ready in about 1 hour | Servings 8)

Ingredients

1. 2 ½ cups dried garbanzo beans, soaked overnight

1. 1/2 cup dry lentils, brown (I have never tried red)

1. 3 ripe tomatoes, diced

1. 1 cup fresh cilantro, finely minced

1. 3 cloves garlic, minced

1. 1 onion, finely chopped

1. 2 carrots, peeled and finely chopped

1. 2 celery ribs, finely chopped

1. 2 tablespoons vegetable oil

1. Sea salt and ground black pepper, to taste

1. 1/4 teaspoon turmeric

1. 1/2 cup flour

1. 3 tablespoons tomato paste

1. 1/2 cup rice noodles

Directions

1. Place garbanzo beans, lentils, tomatoes, and cilantro in your pressurecooker.

2. Add the garlic, onion, carrots, and celery. Pour in enough water to cover thevegetables.

3. Next, add the vegetable oil, salt, black pepper, and turmeric; cover with thelid. Cook for about 15 minutes.

4. In the meantime, combine the flour with 1 cup of warm water. Add thismixture to the cooker along with tomato paste. Cook an additional 10minutes, stirring periodically.

5. Stir in rice noodles and cook for 10 more minutes. Ladle into eight soupbowls and serve warm.

Winter Hearty Chili

(Ready in about 1 hour | Servings 6)

Ingredients

1. 1 ¼ cups pinto beans, soaked for 30 minutes

1. 3 tablespoons canola oil

1. 1 ½ pounds sirloin steaks, cubed

1. 2 cloves garlic, minced

1. 1 leek, chopped

1. 1 tablespoon chili powder

1. 1 bell pepper chopped

1. 3 tomatoes, chopped

1. 1 (28-ounce) can tomato sauce

1. 5 cups beef broth

1. 2 teaspoons sugar

1. Kosher salt and black pepper to taste

Directions

1. Drain and rinse the soaked pinto beans.

2. In the meantime, heat canola oil on HIGH until sizzling. Then, cook thesteak, garlic, and leek for about 5 minutes.

3. Add remaining ingredients; seal the pressure cooker's lid, and set on HIGHfor 24 minutes.

4. Open the lid naturally and adjust your chili for seasonings. Serve warm.

DINNER RECIPES
Delicious Braised Cauliflower
(Ready in about 10 minutes | Servings 6)

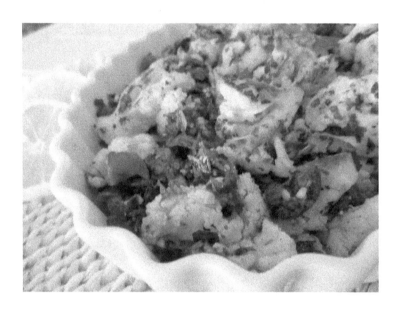

Ingredients

1. 2 tablespoons sesame oil

1. 1/2 cup sweet onion, chopped

1. 2 cloves garlic, crushed

1. 1/4 teaspoon pepper flakes, crushed

1. 1 pound cauliflower, cut into florets

1. 1/2 teaspoon salt

1. 1/4 teaspoon ground black pepper

1. 1/2 teaspoon dried basil

1. 3/4 cups water

Directions

1. Heat sesame oil in your pressure cooker over medium heat. Add sweet onion, garlic, and red pepper flakes; cook, stirring continuously, for about 2minutes. Add the cauliflower florets and continue cooking for about 5 minutes.

2. Sprinkle with salt, black pepper, and dried basil; add the water.

3. Cook for 2 to 3 minutes at HIGH pressure. Lastly, open the cooker byfollowing the manufacturer's instructions. Serve over rice.

Seared Brussels Sprouts

(Ready in about 10 minutes | Servings 6)

Ingredients

1. 2 tablespoons butter, at room temperature

1. 1 pound Brussels sprouts, outer leaves removed and halved

1. 1/4 cup water

1. Salt and ground black pepper, to taste

1. 1 teaspoon red pepper flakes, to taste

Directions

1. Add butter to your pressure cooker and melt it over medium-high heat. When the butter is melted, cook your Brussels sprouts for a few minutes oruntil tender.

2. Add the water, and lock on the lid. Bring to HIGH pressure, and maintainpressure for about 1 minute. Season with salt, black pepper, and red pepperto taste. Serve as a perfect light dinner.

Tangy Red Cabbage

(Ready in about 10 minutes | Servings 4)

Ingredients

1. 2 cloves garlic, minced

1. 1 bunch scallions, sliced

1. 1 chili pepper, finely minced

1. 1/2 cup water

1. 1/4 cup tamari sauce

1. 4 cups red cabbage, cut into strips

1. 2 carrots, julienned

Directions

1. Add the garlic, scallions, chili pepper, water, and tamari sauce to yourpressure cooker; stir well. Stir in the cabbage and carrots.

2. Cover and bring to HIGH pressure; maintain pressure for 2 minutes.

3. Afterwards, remove the lid according to manufacturer's instructions. Transfer to a large platter and serve.

DESSERT RECIPES
Rice Pudding with Cranberries
(Ready in about 30 minutes | Servings 6)

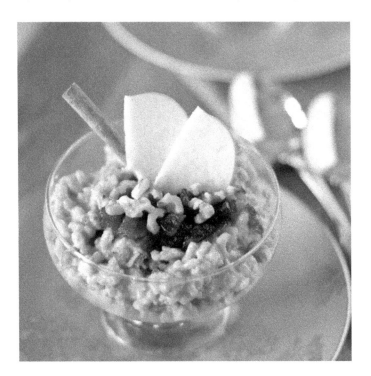

Ingredients

1. 1 ½ cups rice, rinsed and drained

1. 2 cups almond milk

1. 2 cups water

1. 1/2 cup sugar

1. 1/2 teaspoon allspice

1. 1/4 teaspoon cardamom

1. 1/4 teaspoon nutmeg, freshly grated

1. 1/8 teaspoon sea salt

1. 1 cup dried cranberries

Directions

1. Add rice, almond milk, water, sugar, allspice, cardamom, nutmeg, and sea salt to your pressure cooker. Set the cooker over medium-high heat; bringto a boil.

2. Cover with the lid and cook for 15 minutes on LOW pressure.

3. Remove the lid according to manufacturer's instructions. Stir in cranberries.Allow the pudding to sit approximately 15 minutes. Serve and enjoy.

Apple and Dried Cherry Treat

(Ready in about 10 minutes | Servings 10)

Ingredients

1. 4 tart apples, peeled, cored and grated

1. 4 sweet apples peeled, cored and grated

1. 1 cup dried cherries

1. Grated rind and juice from 1 medium-sized orange

1. 1/2 cup brown sugar

1. 1/2 cup granulated sugar

1. 1 tablespoon butter

1. 1/2 teaspoon ground cloves

1. 1/8 teaspoon salt

1. 1/2 teaspoon cardamom

1. 1/2 teaspoon cinnamon

Directions

1. Add the apples and dried cherries to your pressure cooker. Place the remaining ingredients over the fruits.

2. Next, lock the lid into place, and bring to LOW pressure; maintain pressure approximately 5 minutes. Afterwards, allow pressure to release naturally and remove the lid.

3. Stir well and serve at room temperature.

Walnut Butter Cheesecake

(Ready in about 35 minutes | Servings 10)

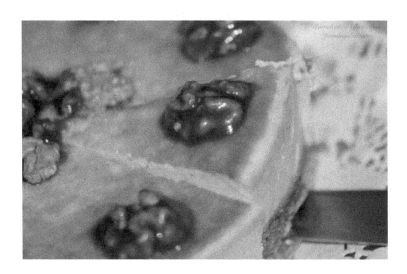

Ingredients

For the Crust:

1. 1/2 cup graham cracker crumbs

1. 1/4 cup walnuts, chopped

1. 2 tablespoons margarine, meltedFor the Filling:

1. 1 pound Ricotta cheese, softened

1. 2/3 cup nut butter

1. 3⁄4 cup granulated sugar

1. 3 eggs

1. 1/4 teaspoon almond extract

1. 3⁄4 teaspoon vanilla extract

Directions

1. Coat two metal cake pans with non-stick cooking spray. Make two crustsby mixing graham cracker crumbs, together with walnuts, and margarine.

2. Process the filling ingredients in your blender or a food processor. Spreadthe filling over the top of each crust.

3. Next, place a metal rack at the bottom of the pressure cooker. To create awater bath, pour 2 cups of water into the bottom of your cooker.

4. Place the cake pans on the metal rack in prepared cooker. Cover with an aluminum foil. Cook for 25 minutes on HIGH. Remove the lid according tomanufacturer's instructions. Place in the refrigerator until chilled.

INSTANT POT

BREAKFAST RECIPES
Creamy Quick Oats
(Ready in about 10 minutes | Servings 4)

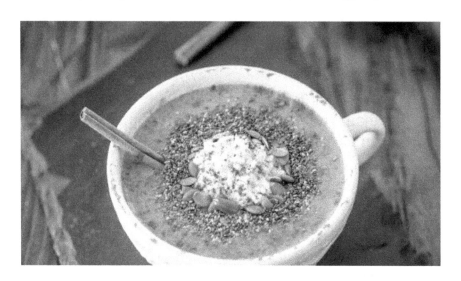

Ingredients

1. 1 cup water

1. 1 cup oats

1. 1 2/3 cups water

1. 2 cups water

1. A pinch of salt

1. A dash of cinnamon

1. Cream, for garnish

Directions

1. Pour 1 cup of water into your Instant Pot; now place the trivet in the pot.

2. Put oats together with 1 2/3 cups of water into a heat-proof bowl; place thebowl on the trivet.

3. Press "Manual" and cook for about 7 minutes. Next, quick release steam.

4. Divide among serving bowls and top with cream. Enjoy!

White Wheat Berries with Potatoes

(Ready in about 15 minutes | Servings 4)

Ingredients

1. 2 cups white wheat berries, soaked overnight in lots of water

1. 2 tablespoons olive oil

1. 2 medium onions, peeled and sliced

1. 3 cloves garlic, smashed

1. 1/2 teaspoon dried rosemary

1. 1/2 teaspoon dried thyme

1. 4 medium potatoes, cubed

Directions

1. Combine white wheat berries and 6 ½ cups water in your Instant Pot.

2. In a sauté pan, warm olive oil over medium-high heat. Then, sauté the onions and garlic until tender. Add rosemary and thyme and cook for 1more minute, stirring frequently.

3. Choose "Multi-grain" setting and cook wheat together with potatoes. Whenthe mixture is cooked, add sautéed onions and garlic. Sprinkle with seasoned salt and ground black pepper. Serve.

Oats with Honey and Walnuts

(Ready in about 10 minutes | Servings 4)

Ingredients

1. 1 cup steel-cut oats

1. 2 cups water

1. 1/8 teaspoon kosher salt

1. 1 tablespoon honey

1. 1/2 teaspoon walnuts, chopped

Directions

1. Add 1 cup of water to your Instant Pot. Place trivet in the pot.

2. Throw steel-cut oats with two cups of water and salt in a heat-proof bowl; place the bowl on the trivet. Lock in cooker's lid. Use "Manual", and cookfor about 6 minutes.

3. While oats are cooking, toast the walnuts in a clean cast-iron skillet.

4. When your oats are ready, add honey and stir to combine. Serve sprinkledwith some chopped walnuts.

Wheat Berry with Veggies and Greek Yogurt

(Ready in about 15 minutes | Servings 4)

Ingredients

1. 2 cups white wheat berries, soaked overnight in lots of water

1. 2 tablespoons butter

1. 2 sweet onions, peeled and sliced

1. Salt and black pepper, to taste

1. 2 medium carrots, thinly sliced

1. 2 celery stalks, chopped

1. Greek yogurt, for garnish

Directions

1. In your Instant Pot, combine white wheat berries with 6 ½ cups water.

2. In a pan, melt the butter over medium heat. Then, sauté sweet onions untiltender and translucent. Add salt and ground black pepper.

3. Press "Multi-grain" setting; cook wheat together with carrots and celeryuntil they are tender. Now add sautéed sweet onions. Serve topped withGreek yogurt.

Congee with Seeds

(Ready in about 45 minutes | Servings 6)

Ingredients

1. 1/2 cup brown rice

1. 1/8 cup peanut, coarsely chopped

1. 1/4 cup walnut, minced

1. 2 tablespoons sesame seeds

1. 1 teaspoon hemp seeds

1. 1/4 cup dates, pitted and chopped

1. 7 cups of water

Directions

1. Simply put all the above ingredients into your Instant Pot.

2. Now press "Congee" button. To serve: divide among six serving bowls; dotwith soy sauce if desired. Enjoy!

LUNCH RECIPES
Rigatoni with Sausage and Bacon
(Ready in about 15 minutes | Servings 4)

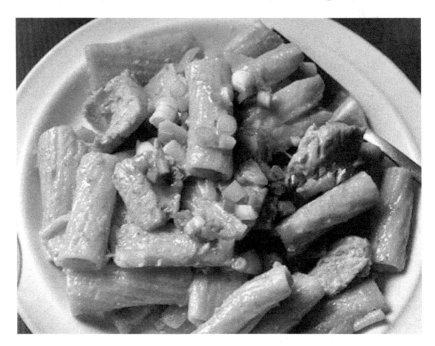

Ingredients

1. 1 tablespoon olive oil

1. 1 cup bacon

1. 1 pound sausage meat

1. 1 medium-sized leek, chopped

1. 2 cloves garlic, peeled and minced

1. 2 cups tomato purée

1. Salt and ground black pepper, to taste

1. 1 teaspoon red pepper flakes crushed

1. 1 pound dry rigatoni pasta

1. 1 tablespoon fresh sage

1. 1 tablespoon fresh basil, chopped

1. 1/4 cup Parmigiano-Reggiano, grated

Directions

1. Press "Sauté" button. Then, warm olive oil. Cook the bacon for about 4minutes. Now, add sausage meat and cook until it is browned and thoroughly cooked.

2. Add the leeks and garlic; sauté them for a few minutes. Now add tomatopurée, salt, black pepper, and red pepper flakes. Add rigatoni pasta and water to cover your pasta.

3. Close and lock the lid. Choose "MANUAL" and LOW pressure for 5 minutes.

4. Afterwards, release the pressure by using the quick pressure release. Stir insage, basil and Parmigiano-Reggiano. Enjoy!

Old-Fashioned Minestrone Soup

(Ready in about 25 minutes | Servings 4)

Ingredients

1. 1 pound ground beef

1. 1 cup cooked beans

1. 1 large-sized potato, diced

1. 2 carrots, trimmed and thinly sliced

1. 2 celery stalks, chopped

1. 1 onion, chopped

1. 3 cloves garlic, minced

1. 32 ounces beef broth

1. 28 ounces canned tomatoes, crushed

1. 1 teaspoon sea salt

1. 1/2 teaspoon ground black pepper

Directions

1. Add the ingredients to your Instant Pot and stir to combine.

2. Put the lid on; choose "MANUAL" and high pressure for 20 minutes. Servewarm and enjoy.

Delicious Short Ribs with Vegetables

(Ready in about 50 minutes | Servings 8)

Ingredients

1. 8 short ribs, excess fat trimmed
1. Sea salt and freshly ground black pepper, to taste
1. 2 tablespoons vegetable oil
1. 1 parsnip, chopped
1. 3 carrots, peeled and thinly sliced
1. 3 cloves garlic, peeled and finely minced
1. 1 red onion, chopped
1. 1 cup vegetable broth
1. 1 cup water
1. 2 tablespoons tomato paste
1. 8 potatoes, small
1. 1 sprig rosemary

1. 1 bay leaf

Directions

1. Generously season the short ribs with sea salt and black pepper. Warm vegetable oil in the inner pot. Push the "MEAT" button. Now brown the ribs on all sides. Reserve the ribs.

2. Add the parsnip, carrots, garlic, and onion; sauté for 4 minutes.

3. Add the reserved browned ribs back to the pot; stir in the rest of the ingredients. Press the "STEW"; then, cook for 40 minutes.

4. Afterwards, remove the lid according to manufacturer's instructions. Serve.

Creamy Potato
Soup

(Ready in about 30 minutes | Servings 6)

Ingredients

1. 8 medium potatoes, peeled and diced

1. 1 celery stalk, thinly sliced

1. 3 carrots, sliced

1. 1/2 cup celery, chopped

1. 1/2 cup spinach leaves, chopped

1. 1 yellow onion, chopped

1. 3 cups broth

1. Salt and ground black pepper, to taste

1. 1 tablespoon fresh basil leaves, finely chopped

1. 1/2 teaspoon red pepper flakes, crushed

1. 1 tablespoon ground f chia seeds

1. Sharp Cheddar cheese, grated

Directions

1. Simply throw all ingredients, except for the cheese, into your Instant Pot.Now press the "Soup" button and adjust the timer to 30 minutes.

2. Process the soup with an immersion blender. Ladle the soup into bowls; topwith grated cheese. Serve with cornbread if desired.

Mushroom and Bean Soup

(Ready in about 25 minutes | Servings 4)

Ingredients

1. 1 pound mushrooms, thinly sliced

1. 1 cup canned cannellini beans

1. 2 carrots, trimmed and thinly sliced

1. 1 large-sized parsnip, chopped

1. 2 celery stalks, chopped

1. 3 cloves garlic, minced

1. 1 onion, chopped

1. 4 cups vegetable stock, preferably homemade

1. 3 cups canned tomatoes, crushed

1. 1/2 teaspoon dried basil

1. 1/2 teaspoon dried dill weed

1. 1 teaspoon sea salt

1. 1/2 teaspoon ground black pepper

Directions

1. Simply throw all ingredients into your Instant Pot; stir to combine well.

2. Cover with the lid and choose "MANUAL" function and "HIGH" pressurefor 20 minutes. Serve right now.

DINNER RECIPES
Peanut and Vegetable Salad
(Ready in about 25 minutes | Servings 4)

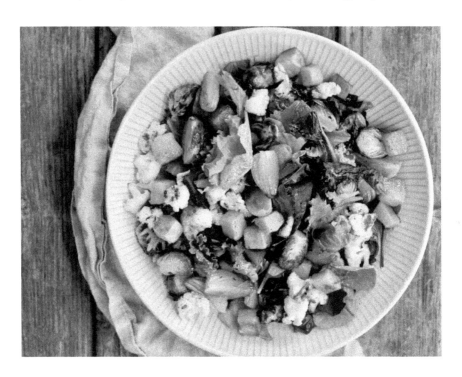

Ingredients

1. 1 pound raw peanuts, shelled

1. 2 cups water

1. 1 bay leaf

1. 2 tomatoes, chopped

1. 1 cup sweet onion, diced

1. 1/4 cup hot peppers, finely minced

1. 1/4 cup celery, diced

1. 2 tablespoons fresh lime juice

1. 2 tablespoons olive oil

1. 3/4 teaspoon salt

1. 1/2 teaspoon freshly ground black pepper

Directions

1. First, blanch raw peanuts in boiling salted water for about 1 minute; drain.Then, discard the skins.

2. Next, cook peanuts, along with two cups of water and the bay leaf; letpeanuts cook about 20 minutes under pressure.

3. Transfer cooked peanuts to a large-sized salad bowl. Add the remainingingredients and toss to combine.

Pulled BBQ Beef

(Ready in about 1 hour 10 minutes |
Servings 6)

Ingredients

1. Non-stick cooking spray

1. 1 1/3 pounds frozen beef roast

    1. *1 bee*f stock For the BBQ sauce:

1. 1/2 cup ketchup

1. 2 teaspoons honey

1. 1 teaspoon paprika

1. 1 teaspoon kosher salt

1. 1/2 teaspoon ground black pepper

1. 1/4 cup water

Directions

1. Oil your Instant Pot with cooking spray. Put beef roast and stock into thepot. Put the lid on, choose the "Meat" key and set to 70 minutes.

2. Meanwhile, combine together the BBQ sauce ingredients in a mixing bowl.

3. Turn the pot off. Next, use a quick pressure release. Now pull the cookedmeat apart into chunks.

4. Add the beef back to the Instant Pot; pour the BBQ sauce over it. Assemblethe sandwiches and serve.

Tuna with Noodles and Feta

(Ready in about 20 minutes | Servings 6)

Ingredients

1. 1 tablespoon vegetable oil

1. 1 red onion, chopped

1. 8 ounces dry egg noodles

1. 1 can (14-ounce) tomatoes, diced

1. 1 ¼ cups water

1. 1 dried basil

1. 1 ½ teaspoons garlic powder

1. 1/2 teaspoon sea salt

1. 1/4 teaspoon black pepper

1. 1 can tuna fish in water, drained

1. Feta cheese, crumbled

Directions

1. Warm the oil and sauté the onion for about 2 minutes.

2. Stir in the noodles, tomatoes, water; click "Soup" button and set time to 10minutes. Turn the pot off.

3. Add the remaining ingredients, except for feta; cook for 4 more minutesuntil it is warmed through. Serve garnished with feta cheese.

Party Barbecue Pork

(Ready in about 1 hour | Servings 16)

Ingredients

1. 8 pounds pork butt roast

1. 1 teaspoon cumin powder

1. 1 teaspoon onion powder

1. 1 teaspoon garlic powder

1. Sea salt and black pepper, to your liking

1. 2 (12-ounce) bottles barbecue sauce

Directions

1. Season the pork with cumin powder, onion powder, garlic powder, salt andblack pepper; now fill the cooker with enough water to cover.

2. Close the lid and press "Meat" button. Cook for 1 hour.

3. Reserve 2 cups of cooking juice. Shred your pork and drizzle with barbecuesauce. Serve right now.

Pasta with Beef and Tomato Sauce

(Ready in about 10 minutes | Servings 6)

Ingredients

1. 1 pound lean ground beef

1. 2 pounds tomato paste

1. 1 onion

1. 2 garlic cloves, minced

1. 1 pound fresh mushrooms, chopped

1. Sea salt and ground black pepper, to taste

1. 1/2 teaspoon dried dill weed

1. 1/2 teaspoon dried basil

1. 1 pound dried egg noodles

Directions

1. Press "Sauté" button and brown the beef.

2. Add the rest of the ingredients. Pressure cook for 7 minutes. Serve warm.

FAST SNACKS
Favorite Steamed Artichokes
(Ready in about 25 minutes | Servings 2)

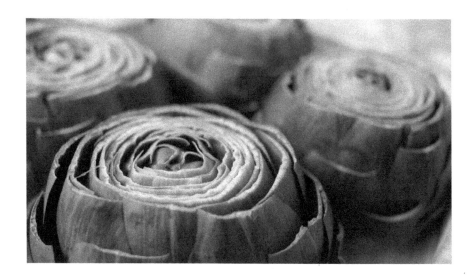

Ingredients

1. 2 whole artichokes

1. 1/2 lime

1. White pepper, to taste

1. 1 cup water

Directions

1. Rinse the artichokes and remove any outer leaves. Now trim off the stem and top third of each artichoke with a sharp knife. Drizzle with lime juice.Sprinkle with white pepper.

2. Set a steamer basket into your cooker. Pour 1 cup of water at the base ofyour cooker. Lay the artichokes in the steamer basket and pour in a cup ofwater.

3. Close the lid. Choose "Manual" function; adjust the time to 20 minutes.Serve with your favorite dipping sauce.

Sweet Baby Carrots

(Ready in about 20 minutes | Servings 6)

Ingredients

1. 1 tablespoon butter

1. 1 tablespoon brown sugar

1. 1/2 cup water

1. 1/4 teaspoon kosher salt

1. 1 pound baby carrots

Directions

1. Put the butter, sugar, water and kosher salt into the Instant Pot. Select "Sauté" key and cook for 30 seconds, stirring continuously. Stir in thecarrots.

2. Put the lid on cooker, select "Steam" key, and set the timer to 15 minutes.

3. Next, uncover and select "Sauté" button. Cook until pot juice has evaporated. Serve.

Marinated Artichoke Appetizer

(Ready in about 15 minutes | Servings 6)

Ingredients

1. 4 large artichokes, trimmed and stems removed

1. 2 tablespoons fresh orange juice

1. 2 teaspoons apple cider vinegar

1. 1/4 cup olive oil

1. 2 cloves garlic, minced fine

1. 1/2 teaspoon dried dill weed

1. 1 teaspoon onion powder

1. 1/2 teaspoon sea salt

1. 1/2 teaspoon fresh ground black pepper

Directions

1. Place steamed basket in your Instant Pot. Arrange the artichokes, bottom up, in a steamer basket; add 2 cups of water.

2. Select the "Steam" setting; set cooking time to 8 minutes.

3. Meanwhile, prepare the marinade. Combine the rest of the ingredients in amixing bowl.

4. Cut cooked artichokes in half. Drizzle the marinade over the warmartichokes. Allow the artichokes to sit overnight.

Honey Chicken Wings

(Ready in about 25 minutes | Servings 5)

Ingredients

1. 10 chicken wings

1. 1 teaspoon shallot powder

1. 1/2 teaspoon coriander

1. 1 teaspoon cumin powder

1. 1 teaspoon garlic powder

1. 1/2 cup honey

1. 1 tablespoon apple cider vinegar

1. Salt and ground black pepper, to your liking

Directions

1. Preheat your oven to 400 degrees F.

2. Place chicken wings in your Instant Pot. Place lid on and select the "POULTRY" setting. Reserve the liquid.

3. Transfer the chicken wings to the oven and roast them until skin is crispy. Remove the chicken from oven and set aside in a baking dish to keep warm.

4. Add the rest of the ingredients to the pot with chicken broth; push "SAUTE" button. Cook for 10 to 15 minutes, stirring continuously. Pourthe sauce over the chicken wings, and serve.

Easy Carrot Snack

(Ready in about 10 minutes | Servings 8)

Ingredients

1. 2 tablespoons butter

1. 1 ½ pounds carrots, cut into matchsticks

1. 1/4 teaspoon baking soda

1. 1/4 cup packed brown sugar

1. A pinch of salt

1. 1/2 teaspoon grated orange peel

Directions

1. Place butter in your Instant Pot. Add the carrots along with the remainingingredients.

2. Pressure cook for 4 minutes. Serve.

DESSERT RECIPES
Black Chocolate Delight
(Ready in about 15 minutes | Servings 6)

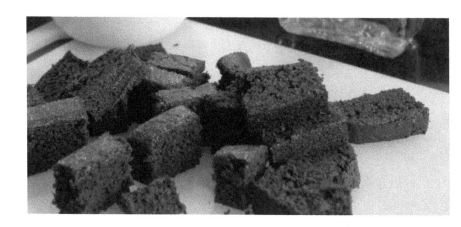

Ingredients

1. 1 ½ cups black chocolate

1. 1 stick butter

1. 3/4 cup brown sugar

1. 1/2 teaspoon vanilla extract

1. 1 teaspoon almond extract

1. 1/4 cup all-purpose flour

1. 3 whole eggs

Directions

1. In a pan, melt chocolate and butter. Add the remaining ingredients and beatwith an electric mixer.

2. Divide the batter among ramekins. Choose "Manual" and cook for 6 minutes. Quick release pressure and allow your cakes to rest for severalminutes before removing from ramekins. Enjoy!

Rice Pudding with Zante Currants

(Ready in about 30 minutes | Servings 6)

Ingredients

1. 1 ½ cups Arborio rice

1. A pinch of salt

1. 3/4 cups sugar

1. 5 cups milk

1. 2 eggs

1. 1 cup half and half

1. 1/2 teaspoon ground cinnamon

1. 1/4 teaspoon grated nutmeg

1. 1/2 teaspoon almond extract

1. 1/2 teaspoon vanilla extract

1. 1 cup Zante currants

Directions

1. In the inner pot, combine, rice, salt, sugar, and milk.

2. Select the "Sauté" mode. Bring to a boil, stirring constantly, until sugar isdissolved. Then, cover and select the "Rice" mode.

3. In the meantime, in a mixing bowl, whisk the eggs, half and half, cinnamon,nutmeg, almond extract, and the vanilla extract.

4. When you hear the beep sound, press "Cancel". Wait 15 minutes, and perform the quick pressure release. While the mixture is still hot, stir in theegg mixture. Now add Zante currants and stir to combine.

5. Press the "Sauté" key. Cook until the mixture begins to boil. Then, turn offthe cooker. Serve at room temperature.

Sweet Peach and Coconut Risotto

(Ready in about 20 minutes | Servings 6)

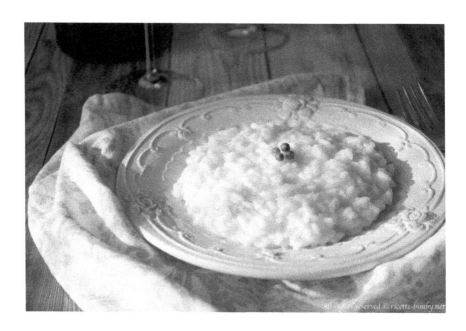

Ingredients

1. 2 ripe peaches, pitted and halved

1. 4 cups coconut milk

1. Zest and juice of 1 orange

1. 1 ¾ cups rice

1. 1/2 teaspoon vanilla extract

1. 1/2 cup coconut flakes

1. 1/4 teaspoon nutmeg, preferably freshly grated

1. 1/4 cup candied ginger, diced

Directions

1. Place all the above ingredients in your cooker.

2. Choose "Manual" mode; set time to 12 minutes. Serve garnished with whipped cream if desired.

CPSIA information can be obtained
at www.ICGtesting.com
Printed in the USA
BVHW090303180521
607554BV00009B/2115